Length Tension Testing Book 1, Lower Quadrant

A WORKBOOK OF MANUAL THERAPY TECHNIQUES

SECOND EDITION

Paolo Sanzo, DScPT, MSc, BScPT, FCAMT
Murray MacHutchon, BMRPT, FCAMT

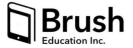 **Brush**
Education Inc.

Brush Education Inc.
www.brusheducation.ca
contact@brusheducation.ca

Photographer: Allan Dickson Photography
Model: Melinda Vaillant
Cover design: Dean Pickup
Interior design: Carol Dragich, Dragich Design

Printed and manufactured in Canada

Library and Archives Canada Cataloguing in Publication
Sanzo, Paolo, 1969–, author
Length tension testing : a workbook of manual therapy techniques /
Paolo Sanzo, DScPT, MSC, BSCPT, FCAMT, Murray MacHutchon,
BMRPT, FCAMT. — Second edition.

Originally published in 2007. Includes bibliographical references.
Contents: Book 1. Lower quadrant Issued in print and electronic formats.
ISBN 978-1-55059-592-5 (pbk. : bk. 1).—ISBN 978-1-55059-593-2 (pdf : bk. 1).—
ISBN 978-1-55059-594-9 (mobi : bk. 1).—ISBN 978-1-55059-595-6 (epub : bk. 1).

1. Physical therapy.   I. MacHutchon, Murray, author   II. Title.

RM700.S36 2015   615.8′2   C2014-907343-7
                                         C2014-907344-5

We also acknowledge the financial support of the Government of Canada through the Canada Book Fund for our publishing activities.

Acknowledgements

Together we are thankful for all the dedicated and hard-working physiotherapists who have volunteered countless hours to make the Orthopaedic Division of the Canadian Physiotherapy Association a success and recognized all over the world.

We are also thankful to our ever-loving families who are supportive in all of our endeavors.

Contents

Introduction

Assessment

The assessment of length tension in muscle involves the use of clinical reasoning and interpretation of the subjective and objective assessment findings. These findings include:

- the referral pattern of pain;
- positional findings on observation;
- changes in active and passive range of motion;
- findings on palpation; and
- activation of the muscle and the flexibility of the muscle during the length tension assessment of the myofascial structures.

Differentiation must also be made in the tension and barrier that are palpated to determine whether this is due to the myofascial tissue or the neuromeningeal tissue. Conclusions are then based on these combined tests and the muscle is determined to be normal, hypertonic, shortened or lengthened.

The therapist may incorporate principles of neuromeningeal assessment to determine whether the tension and barrier present are due to the myofascial tissues or to the neuromeningeal structures. Excellent resources are available on the assessment of neuromeningeal tissue, and readers are advised to refer to these for further information and more details. Therapists must have an appreciation for the uniqueness of our anatomy. All tension testing described in this book may have to be slightly altered to accommodate the examiner's or the patient's anatomy.

End feel

The different sensations imparted to the hand of the therapist at the extremes of the passive range of motion is termed the *end feel*. The end feel caused by changes in the myofascial system will be different from some of the end feels associated with a joint restriction.

Normal muscle at rest, and preferably with gravity eliminated, will feel soft. It will have the same feel as palpating raw steak or soft tofu. The length and tension will be as expected for the age of the patient. The contralateral muscle can be tested to confirm this. A normal muscle will contract with voluntary electromyographic (EMG) activity.

Hypertonic muscle has increased elastic and viscoelastic stiffness in the absence of contractile activity. Palpation of the hypertonic muscle will feel similar to palpating well-done steak, and it will have decreased length on testing. Muscle spasm is an abnormal muscle contraction and is often painful. The EMG activity is not under voluntary control. This strong contraction will limit movement significantly. A muscle spasm is velocity dependent. If the muscle is lengthened or moved quickly, spasm will increase.

Truly shortened muscle, or a muscle contracture, is often present post trauma and will feel gristly, tight and short on testing. The muscle contractile unit is shortened in the absence of EMG activity. When the muscle is lengthened or moved, the response is velocity independent. It does not matter if the movement is performed quickly or slowly, the response and length remains unchanged.

The therapist must recognize the different sensations imparted to the hands at the end of the available passive range of motion and gently sense the point at which the range of motion stops. It is with our palpation skills that we determine that it is in fact the muscle being tested that is felt to be tense and that is providing the resistance to the passive movement. Both the hand providing stabilization and the hand moving the body part must together sense the tension in the muscle and the barrier present.

Clinical reasoning
Length tension test findings may be unrelated to the palpation findings found in muscle at rest. Therapists must base their conclusions on a clinical reasoning approach to rule out other problems or tissues at fault. Length tension testing should preferably be performed in supine lying or prone lying to unload the muscle and neutralize the effect of gravity. This cannot always be done, however, and thus alternative test positions are also described.

Disclaimer

The procedures described in this book should be implemented in a manner consistent with professional standards set for the circumstances that apply in each situation. Every effort has been made to confirm accuracy of the information presented and to correctly relate generally accepted practices.

Nevertheless, practitioners must always rely on their own experience, knowledge, and judgment when consulting any of the information contained in this reference or employing it in patient care. When using any of this information, they should remain conscious of their responsibility for their own safety and the safety of others, and for the best interests of those in their care.

To the fullest extent of the law, neither the publishers, the authors, nor the editors assume any liability for injury or damage to persons or property from any use of information or ideas contained in this reference.

THE LUMBAR SPINE
AND PELVIS

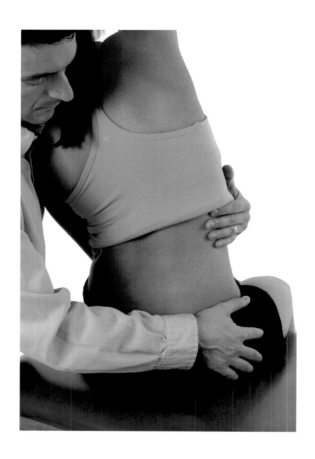

Latissimus Dorsi

Technique 1

Technique described for the bilateral latissimus dorsi muscle.

Patient: Positioned in supine lying with the arms flexed and externally rotated overhead.

Therapist: Standing at the side of the bed observing the lordosis in the lumbar spine.

Action: Note the amount of flexion that occurs in the arms before the lumbar spine lordosis begins to increase. Apply over pressure to the arms at the end of flexion when the lumbar spine lordosis begins to increase. Assess the amount of range and the end feel and note the reproduction of any symptoms.

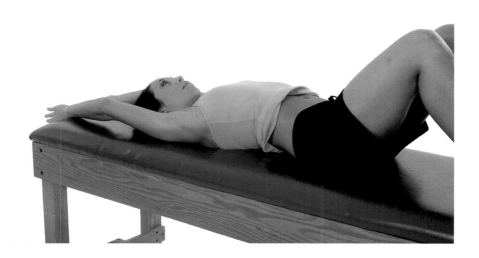

Latissimus Dorsi

Technique 2
Technique described for the right latissimus dorsi
muscle.

Patient: Positioned in left side lying over a pillow that is
  placed in the mid-thoracic spine region.

Therapist: Standing in front of the patient.

Action: Flex and externally rotate the right arm and
  note the amount of flexion that occurs before the
  lumbar spine starts to increase its lordosis. Stabilize
  the innominate and apply over pressure to the right
  arm at the end of flexion and external rotation. Both
  the stabilizing hand and the hand moving the body
  part sense the tension in the muscle and the barrier.
  Assess the amount of range, the end feel and where
  the lumbar spine lordosis begins to increase, and
  note the reproduction of any symptoms. This test is
  then repeated in right side lying and the findings
  compared.

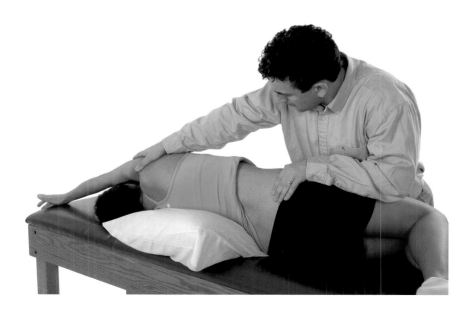

Latissimus Dorsi

Technique 3
Technique described for the right latissimus dorsi
muscle.

Patient: Positioned in standing with the elbows
extended and the arms externally rotated and
adducted.

Therapist: Standing behind the patient and observing
the lumbar spine region.

Action: Horizontally abduct the arms maximally to the
left and note the amount of abduction that occurs
before the lumbar spine lordosis begins to increase.
Assess the amount of range and note the reproduction of any symptoms. Repeat this test with the arms
horizontally abducted to the right and
compare the findings.

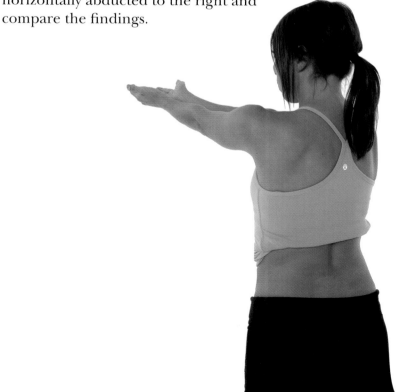

Quadratus Lumborum

Technique 1 – Longitudinal Fibers
Technique described for the right quadratus lumborum muscle.

Patient: Positioned in left side lying over a pillow, with the pillow positioned in the lumbar spine region.

Therapist: Standing in front of the patient.

Action: While stabilizing the patient's right lower two ribs with your right hand, use your left hand to side flex their lumbar spine to the left (toward the floor via the superior aspect of the innominate bone). Both the stabilizing hand and the hand moving the body part sense the tension in the muscle and the barrier. Assess the amount of range and the end feel and note the reproduction of any symptoms. Repeat this test on the contralateral side and compare the two results.

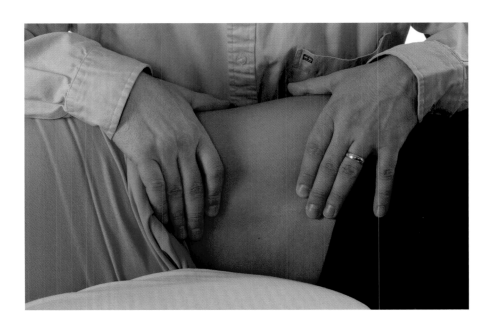

Quadratus Lumborum

Technique 2 – Oblique Fibers
Technique described for the right quadratus lumborum muscle.

Patient: Positioned in left side lying over a pillow, with the pillow positioned in the lumbar spine region.

Therapist: Standing in front of the patient.

Action: Stabilize the patient's right innominate with your left hand, and use your right hand to stabilize their right lower two ribs. The thoracolumbar junction is left side flexed and right rotated to bias the oblique fibers of the right quadratus lumborum muscle. Both the stabilizing hand and the hand moving the body part sense the tension in the muscle and the barrier. Assess the amount of range and the end feel and note the reproduction of any symptoms. Repeat this test on the contralateral side and compare the two results.

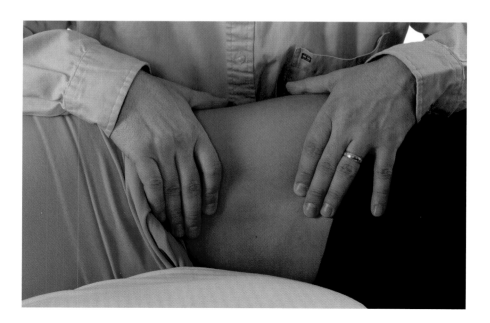

Quadratus Lumborum

Technique 3 – Longitudinal Fibers
Technique described for the right quadratus lumborum muscle.

Patient: Positioned in sitting with the right shoulder girdle maximally flexed and horizontally adducted overhead.

Therapist: Standing to the left side of the patient.

Action: With your right hand, stabilize the right innominate on the bed. With your left hand, side flex the thoracolumbar junction to the left side and add left rotation of the trunk to bias the longitudinal fibers of the right quadratus lumborum muscle. Both the stabilizing hand and the hand moving the body part sense the tension in the muscle and the barrier. Assess the amount of range and the end feel and note the reproduction of any symptoms. Repeat this test on the contralateral side and compare the two results.

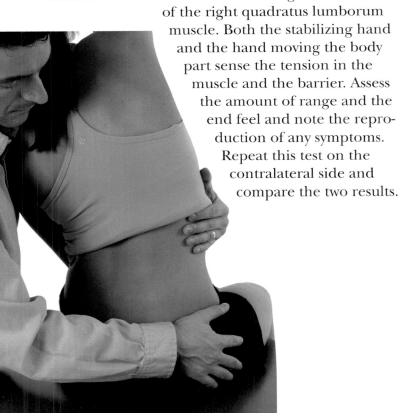

Erector Spinae

Technique 1

Technique described for the bilateral erector spinae muscles.

Patient: Positioned in side lying.

Therapist: Standing in front of the patient.

Action: Stabilize the ribs with your right hand. Use your left hand to maximally flex the thoracic and lumbar spine regions via the hips and innominates to bias the erector spinae muscles bilaterally. Both the stabilizing hand and the hand moving the body part sense the tension in the muscle and the barrier. Assess the amount of range and the end feel and note the reproduction of any symptoms. Repeat this test on the contralateral side and compare the two results.

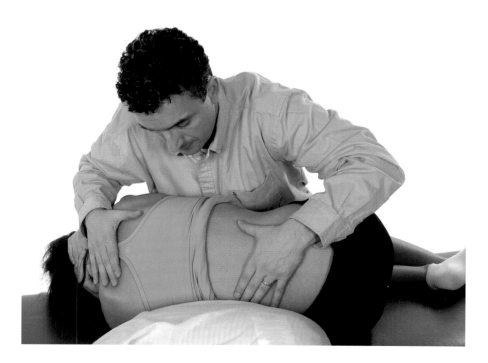

Erector Spinae

Technique 2

Technique described for the right erector spinae muscles.

Patient: Positioned in left side lying with the right shoulder girdle maximally flexed and horizontally adducted overhead and a towel roll or pillow positioned under the left side of the lumbar spine.

Therapist: Standing in front of the patient.

Action: Stabilize the right ribs with your right hand. With your left hand and forearm, maximally flex the thoracic and lumbar spine regions via the right hip and innominate. Add left side flexion of the trunk via the innominate to bias the right erector spinae musculature. Both the stabilizing hand and the hand moving the body part sense the tension in the muscle and the barrier. Assess the amount of range and the end feel and note the reproduction of any symptoms. Repeat this test on the contralateral side and compare the two results.

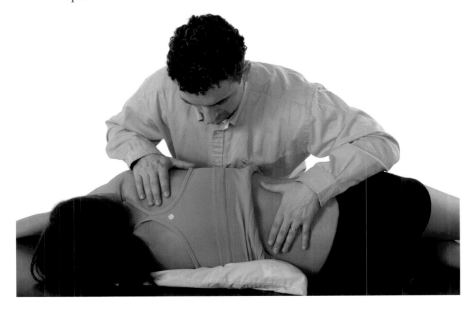

Thoracodorsal Fascia Functional Length Tension Test

Technique 1
Technique described for the right thoracodorsal fascia.

Patient: Positioned in sitting with the lumbar spine in a neutral position and the arms resting by the sides.

Therapist: Standing behind the patient.

Action: Instruct the patient to rotate their trunk to the left. Assess the amount of range and the end feel and note the reproduction of any symptoms. Repeat this test on the contralateral side and compare the two results.

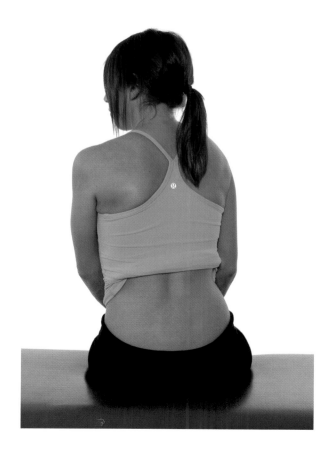

Thoracodorsal Fascia Functional Length Tension Test

Technique 2
Technique described for the right thoracodorsal fascia.

Patient: Positioned in sitting with the lumbar spine in a
neutral position and the arms resting by the sides.

Therapist: Standing behind the patient.

Action: Instruct the patient to flex their arms to 90°
and internally rotate and adduct their shoulders.
Then ask the patient to rotate their trunk to the left.
Assess the amount of range and the end feel and
note the reproduction of any symptoms. Repeat this
test on the contralateral side and compare the two
results.

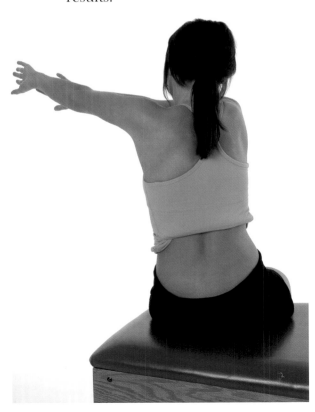

Thoracodorsal Fascia Functional Length Tension Test

Technique 3

Technique described for the right thoracodorsal fascia.

Patient: Positioned in sitting with the lumbar spine in a neutral position and the arms resting by the sides.

Therapist: Standing behind the patient.

Action: Instruct the patient to flex their arms to 90° and externally rotate and adduct their shoulders. Then ask the patient to rotate their trunk to the left. This latter position increases the tension through the latissimus dorsi and the thoracodorsal fascia. Assess the amount of range and the end feel and note the reproduction of any symptoms. Repeat this test on the contralateral side and compare the two results.

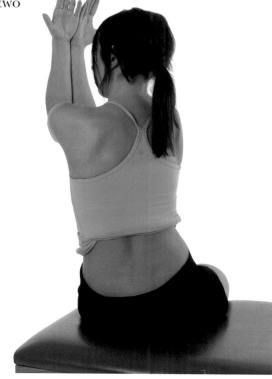

THE HIP

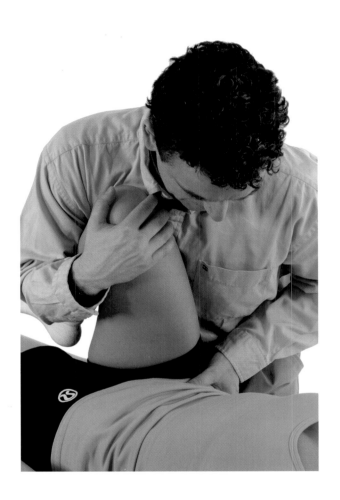

Pectineus

Technique 1
Technique described for the right pectineus muscle.

Patient: Positioned in sitting at the edge of the bed.

Therapist: Standing at the side of the bed.

Action: Position the palmar aspect of your left hand over the patient's right superior pubic ramus. Your right hand supports the proximal aspect of the right femur. Extend and abduct the hip in sitting. Both the stabilizing hand and the hand moving the body part sense the tension in the muscle and the barrier. Assess the amount of range and the end feel and note the reproduction of any symptoms. Repeat this test on the contralateral side and compare the two results.

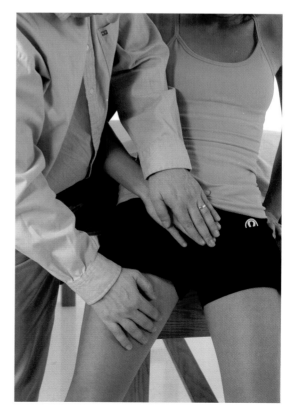

Pectineus

Technique 2
Technique described for the right pectineus muscle.

Patient: Positioned in supine lying at the edge of the
 bed.

Therapist: Standing at the side of the bed.

Action: Position the palmar aspect of your right hand
 over the patient's right superior pubic ramus. Your
 left hand supports the proximal aspect of the right
 femur. Extend and abduct the hip. Both the stabilizing hand and the hand moving the body part sense
 the tension in the muscle and the barrier. Assess
 the amount of range and the end feel and note the
 reproduction of any symptoms. Repeat this test on
 the contralateral side and compare the two results.

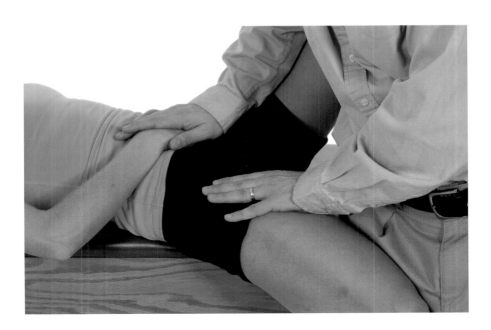

Adductor Longus and Adductor Brevis

Technique described for the right adductor longus and the right adductor brevis muscles.

Patient: Positioned in supine lying.

Therapist: Standing at the side of the bed.

Action: Position the palmar aspect of your left hand lateral to the patient's right superior pubic ramus. Your right hand supports the distal and medial aspect of the right femur. Abduct the hip in neutral. Both the stabilizing hand and the hand moving the body part sense the tension in the muscle and the barrier. Assess the amount of range and the end feel and note the reproduction of any symptoms. Repeat this test on the contralateral side and compare the two results.

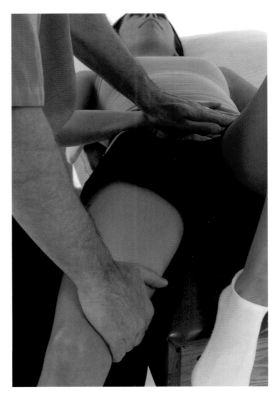

Gracilis

Technique described for the right gracilis muscle.

Patient: Positioned in supine lying.

Therapist: Standing at the side of the bed.

Action: Position the palmar aspect of your left hand lateral to the patient's right superior pubic ramus. Your right hand supports the proximal aspect of the right tibia and fibula distal to the right knee joint.

The hip is extended and abducted and the tibia is externally rotated. Both the stabilizing hand and the hand moving the body part sense the tension in the muscle and the barrier. Assess the amount of range and the end feel of the right hip and note the reproduction of any symptoms. Repeat this test on the contralateral side and compare the two results.

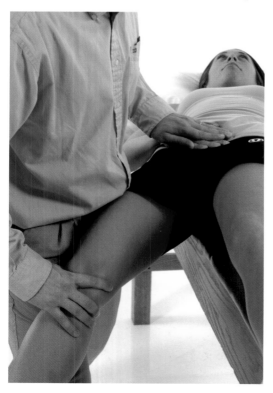

Adductor Magnus (Anterior Fibers)

Technique 1
Technique described for the right adductor magnus muscle.

Patient: Positioned in supine lying at the side of the bed.

Therapist: Standing at the side of the bed.

Action: Position the palmar aspect of your left hand lateral to the patient's right superior pubic ramus. Your right hand supports the distal and medial aspect of the right femur proximal to the right knee joint. Extend and abduct the hip in supine lying to bias the anterior fibers of the adductor magnus muscle. Both the stabilizing hand and the hand moving the body part sense the tension in the muscle and the barrier. Assess the amount of range and the end feel and note the reproduction of any symptoms. Repeat this test on the contralateral side and compare the two results.

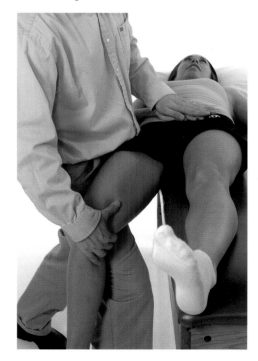

Adductor Magnus (Anterior Fibers)

Technique 2
Technique described for the right adductor magnus
muscle.

Patient: Positioned in left side lying.

Therapist: Standing behind the patient.

Action: Position the palmar aspect of your left hand
   lateral to the patient's right superior pubic ramus.
   Your right hand supports the distal and medial
   aspect of the right femur with the right knee flexed.
   Extend and abduct the hip in side lying to bias the
   anterior fibers of the adductor magnus muscle. Both
   the stabilizing hand and the hand moving the body
   part sense the tension in the muscle and the barrier.
   Assess the amount of range and the end feel and
   note the reproduction of any symptoms. Repeat this
   test on the contralateral side and compare the two
   results.

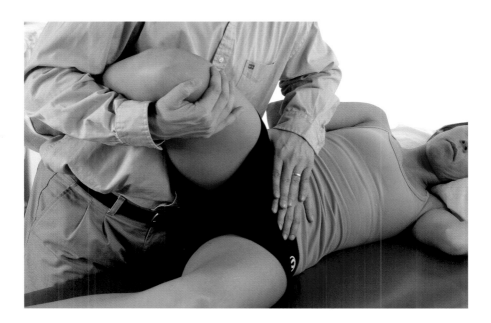

Adductor Magnus (Posterior Fibers)

Technique 1

Technique described for the right adductor magnus muscle.

Patient: Positioned in supine lying at the side of the bed for the posterior fibers.

Therapist: Standing at the side of the bed.

Action: Position the palmar aspect of your left hand lateral to the patient's right superior pubic ramus. Your right hand supports the distal aspect of the right femur proximal to the right knee joint with the right knee flexed. Flex and abduct the hip in supine lying to bias the posterior fibers of the adductor magnus muscle. Both the stabilizing hand and the hand moving the body part sense the tension in the muscle and the barrier. Assess the amount of range and the end feel of the right hip and note the reproduction of any symptoms. Repeat this test on the contralateral side and compare the two results.

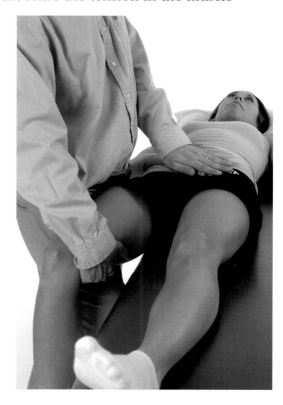

Adductor Magnus (Posterior Fibers)

Technique 2
Technique described for the right adductor magnus
muscle.

Patient: Positioned in left side lying for the posterior
fibers.

Therapist: Standing at the side of the bed.

Action: Position the palmar aspect of your left hand lateral to the patient's right superior pubic ramus. Your
right hand supports the distal and medial aspect of
the right femur with the right knee flexed. Flex and
abduct the hip in side lying to bias the posterior
fibers of the adductor magnus muscle. Both the stabilizing hand and the hand moving the body part sense
the tension in the muscle and the barrier. Assess the
amount of range and the end feel of the right hip
and note the reproduction of any symptoms. Repeat
this test on the contralateral side and compare the
two results.

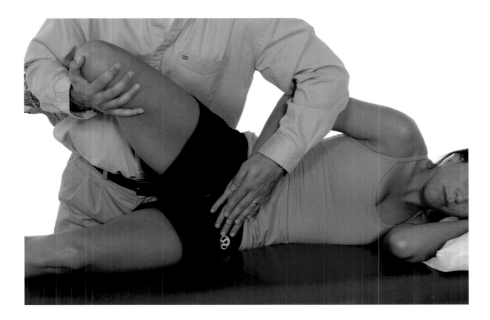

Medial Rotators of the Hip

Technique 1
Technique described for the right hip medial rotators.

Patient: Positioned in supine lying with the right hip flexed to 90° and the right knee flexed to 90°.

Therapist: Standing at the side of the bed.

Action: Stabilize the patient's right innominate with your left hand. With your right hand and forearm, support the distal aspect of their right femur and the proximal aspect of their right tibia and fibula. Also stabilize the patient's right leg against the anterior aspect of your own body. Laterally rotate the right hip and assess the amount of range and the end feel of it. Both the stabilizing hand and the hand moving the body part sense the tension in the muscle and the barrier. Note the reproduction of any symptoms. Repeat this test on the contralateral side and compare the two results.

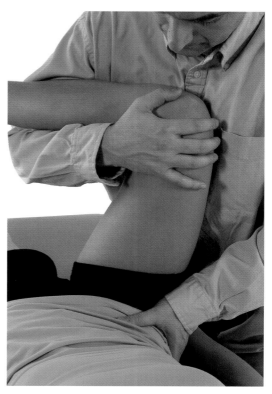

Medial Rotators of the Hip

Technique 2
Technique described for the right hip medial rotators.

Patient: Positioned in supine lying with the right hip in neutral and the right knee fully extended.

Therapist: Standing at the side of the bed.

Action: Stabilize the patient's right innominate with your left hand and support the distal aspect of their right tibia and fibula with your right hand. Laterally rotate the right hip and assess the amount of range and the end feel. Both the stabilizing hand and the hand moving the body part sense the tension in the muscle and the barrier. Note the reproduction of any symptoms. Repeat this test on the contralateral side and compare the two results.

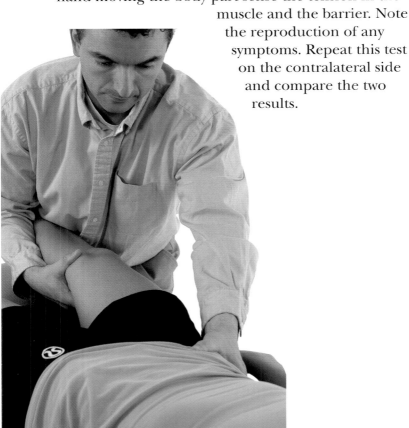

Medial Rotators of the Hip

Technique 3
Technique described for the right hip medial rotators.

Patient: Positioned in prone lying with the right hip in neutral and the right knee flexed to 90°.

Therapist: Standing at the side of the bed.

Action: Stabilize the posterior aspect of the patient's right innominate with your left hand and support the distal aspect of their right tibia and fibula with your right hand. Laterally rotate the right hip and assess the amount of range and the end feel. Both the stabilizing hand and the hand moving the body part sense the tension in the muscle and the barrier. Note the reproduction of any symptoms. Repeat this test on the contralateral side and compare the two results.

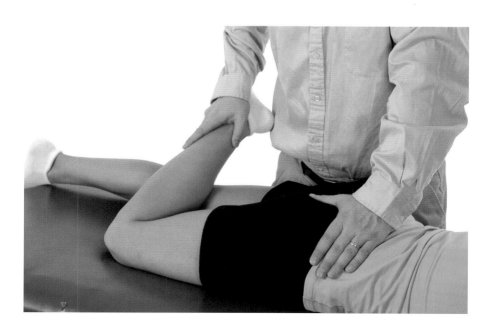

Medial Rotators of the Hip

Technique 4
Technique described for the right hip medial rotators.

Patient: Positioned in prone lying with the right hip in neutral and the right knee fully extended.

Therapist: Standing at the side of the bed.

Action: Stabilize the posterior aspect of the patient's right innominate with your left hand and support the distal aspect of their right femur with your right hand. Laterally rotate the right hip and assess the amount of range and the end feel. Both the stabilizing hand and the hand moving the body part sense the tension in the muscle and the barrier. Note the reproduction of any symptoms. Repeat this test on the contralateral side and compare the two results.

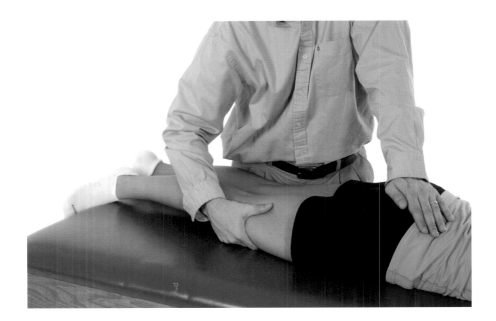

Lateral Rotators of the Hip

Technique 1
Technique described for the right hip lateral rotators.

Patient: Positioned in supine lying with the right hip flexed to 90° and the right knee flexed to 90°.

Therapist: Standing at the right side of the bed.

Action: Stabilize the patient's right innominate with your left hand. With your right hand, support the distal aspect of the patient's right femur and the proximal aspect of their right tibia and fibula. Also stabilize their right leg against the anterior aspect of your own body. Medially rotate the right hip and assess the amount of range and the end feel. Both the stabilizing hand and the hand moving the body part sense the tension in the muscle and the barrier. Note the reproduction of any symptoms. Repeat this test on the contralateral side and compare the two results.

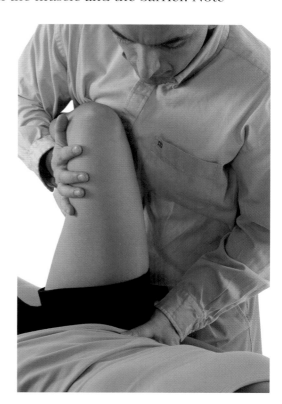

Lateral Rotators of the Hip

Technique 2
Technique described for the right hip lateral rotators.

Patient: Positioned in supine lying with the right hip in neutral and the right knee fully extended.

Therapist: Standing at the right side of the bed.

Action: Stabilize the patient's right innominate with your left hand and support the distal aspect of their right femur, tibia and fibula with your right hand. Medially rotate the right hip and assess the amount of range and the end feel. Both the stabilizing hand and the hand moving the body part sense the tension in the muscle and the barrier. Note the reproduction of any symptoms. Repeat this test on the contralateral side and compare the two results.

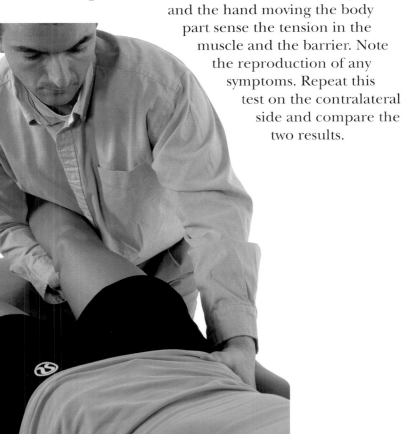

Lateral Rotators of the Hip

Technique 3

Technique described for the right hip lateral rotators.

Patient: Positioned in prone lying with the right hip in neutral and the right knee flexed to 90°.

Therapist: Standing at the side of the bed.

Action: Stabilize the posterior aspect of the patient's right innominate with your left hand and support the distal aspect of their right tibia and fibula with your right hand. Medially rotate the right hip and assess the amount of range and the end feel. Both the stabilizing hand and the hand moving the body part sense the tension in the muscle and the barrier. Note the reproduction of any symptoms. Repeat this test on the contralateral side and compare the two results.

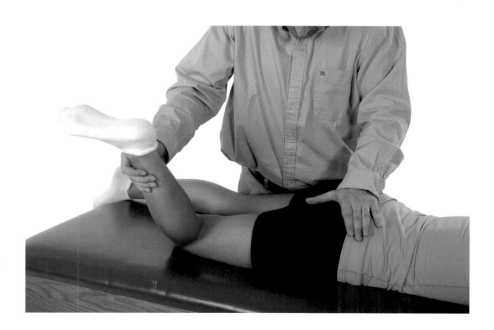

Lateral Rotators of the Hip

Technique 4
Technique described for the right hip lateral rotators.

Patient: Positioned in prone lying with the right hip in neutral and the right knee fully extended.

Therapist: Standing at the right side of the bed.

Action: Stabilize the posterior aspect of the patient's right innominate with your left hand and support the distal aspect of their right tibia and fibula with your right hand. Medially rotate the right hip and assess the amount of range and the end feel. Both the stabilizing hand and the hand moving the body part sense the tension in the muscle and the barrier. Note the reproduction of any symptoms. Repeat this test on the contralateral side and compare the two results.

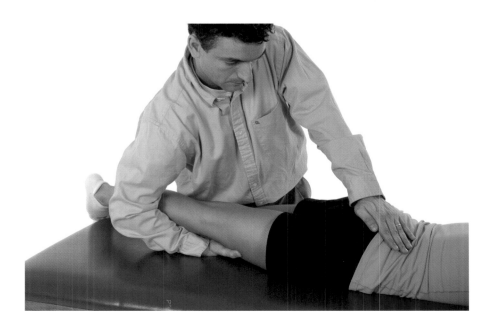

Obturator Externus

Technique described for the right obturator externus muscle.

Patient: Positioned in supine lying.

Therapist: Standing at the side of the bed.

Action: Stabilize the patient's right innominate with your left hand and support the distal aspect of their right tibia and fibula with your right hand. Abduct and medially rotate the right hip and assess the amount of range and the end feel. Both the stabilizing hand and the hand moving the body part sense the tension in the muscle and the barrier. Note the reproduction of any symptoms. Repeat this test on the contralateral side and compare the two results.

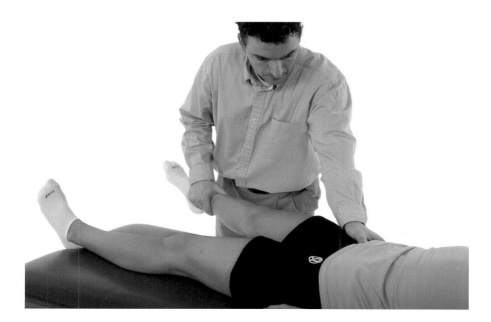

Obturator Internus

Technique described for the right obturator internus muscle.

Patient: Positioned in prone lying.

Therapist: Standing at the side the bed.

Action: Stabilize the posterior aspect of the patient's right innominate with your left hand and support the distal aspect of their right tibia and fibula with your right hand. Extend, adduct and medially rotate the right hip and assess the amount of range and the end feel. Both the stabilizing hand and the hand moving the body part sense the tension in the muscle and the barrier. Note the reproduction of any symptoms. Repeat this test on the contralateral side and compare the two results.

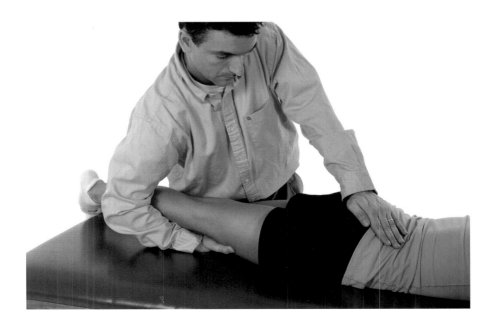

Quadratus Femoris

Technique 1

Technique described for the right quadratus femoris muscle.

Patient: Positioned in supine lying with the right hip in neutral and the right knee fully extended.

Therapist: Standing at the side of the bed.

Action: Stabilize the patient's right innominate with your left hand and support the distal aspect of their right femur, tibia and fibula with your right hand. Medially rotate the right hip and assess the amount of range and the end feel. Both the stabilizing hand and the hand moving the body part sense the tension in the muscle and the barrier. Note the reproduction of any symptoms. Repeat this test on the contra-lateral side and compare the two results.

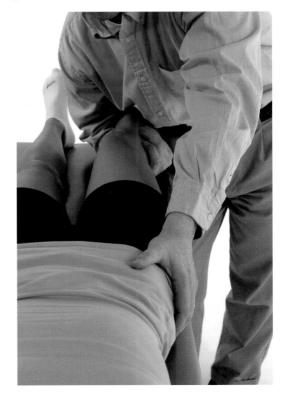

Quadratus Femoris

Technique 2
Technique described for the right quadratus femoris
muscle.

Patient: Positioned in prone lying with the right knee
   flexed to 90°.

Therapist: Standing at the side of the bed.

Action: Stabilize and palpate the lateral aspect of the
   patient's right ischial tuberosity with your left hand.
   With your right hand, palpate the posterior aspect of
   the right greater trochanter and medially rotate the
                              femur. Assess the amount of range
                              and the end feel of the right hip.
                              Both the stabilizing hand and
                              the hand moving the body part
                              sense the tension in the muscle
                              and the barrier. Note the
                              reproduction of any symp-
                              toms. Repeat this test on the
                              contralateral side and com-
                              pare the two results.

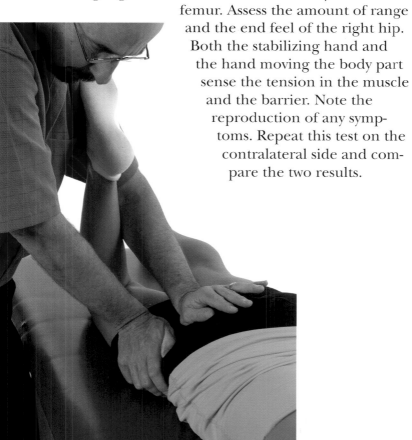

Quadratus Femoris

Technique 3

Technique described for the right quadratus femoris muscle.

Patient: Positioned in prone lying with the right hip internally rotated and the right knee fully extended.

Therapist: Standing at the side of the bed.

Action: Stabilize and palpate the lateral aspect of the patient's right ischial tuberosity with your left hand. With your right hand, palpate the posterior aspect of the right greater trochanter and medially rotate the femur. Assess the amount of range and the end feel of the right hip. Both the stabilizing hand and the hand moving the body part sense the tension in the muscle and the barrier. Note the reproduction of any symptoms. Repeat this test on the contralateral side and compare the two results.

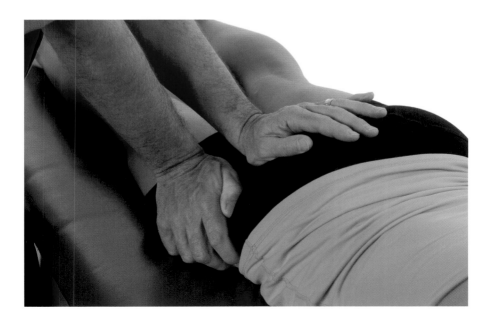

Gluteus Maximus

Technique described for the right gluteus maximus muscle.

Patient: Positioned in supine lying

Therapist: Standing at the side of the bed.

Action: Stabilize the patient's right innominate with your left hand and support their right tibia and fibula with your right hand and forearm. Flex the right hip and right knee and assess the amount of range and the end feel of the right hip. Both the stabilizing hand and the hand moving the body part sense the tension in the muscle and the barrier. Note the reproduction of any symptoms. Repeat this test on the contralateral side and compare the two results.

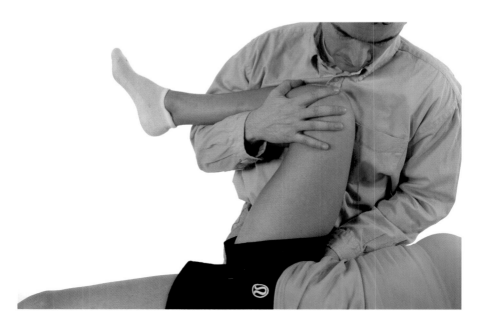

Gluteus Medius (Anterior Fibers) and Gluteus Minimus

Technique described for the right gluteus medius muscle (anterior fibers) and the right gluteus minimus muscle.

Patient: Positioned in prone lying.

Therapist: Standing at the side of the bed.

Action: Stabilize the posterior aspect of the patient's right innominate and sacrum with your left hand and support the distal aspect of their right femur with your right hand and forearm. Adduct, laterally rotate and extend the right hip and assess the amount of range and the end feel. Both the stabilizing hand and the hand moving the body part sense the tension in the muscle and the barrier. Note the reproduction of any symptoms. Repeat this test on the contralateral side and compare the two results.

The actions of the gluteus medius (anterior fibers) and the gluteus minimus muscles are similar to the action of the tensor fascia latae muscle. To bias the gluteus medius (anterior fibers) and the gluteus minimus muscles, take up the adduction component of the combined movements first.

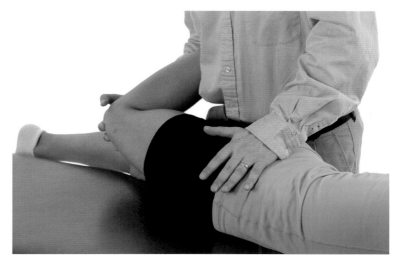

Gluteus Medius (Posterior Fibers)

Technique described for the right gluteus medius muscle (posterior fibers).

Patient: Positioned in supine lying.

Therapist: Standing at the side of the bed on the ipsilateral side.

Action: Stabilize the patient's right innominate with your left hand and support the distal aspect of their right femur with your right hand. Flex the right knee, and flex, adduct and medially rotate the right hip. Assess the amount of range and the end feel of the right hip. Both the stabilizing hand and the hand moving the body part sense the tension in the muscle and the barrier. Note the reproduction of any symptoms. Repeat this test on the contralateral side and compare the two results.

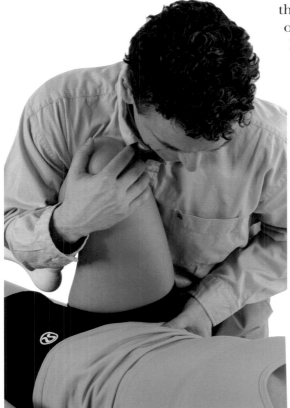

Piriformis

Technique 1

Technique described for the right piriformis muscle.

Patient: Positioned in supine lying with the right knee flexed to 45° to 90°.

Therapist: Standing at the side of the bed on the contralateral side.

Action: Stabilize the patient's right innominate with your right hand and support the lateral aspect of their flexed right knee with your left hand. Adduct and medially rotate the right hip and assess the amount of range and the end feel. Both the stabilizing hand and the hand moving the body part sense the tension in the muscle and the barrier. Note the reproduction of any symptoms. Repeat this test on the contralateral side and compare the two results.

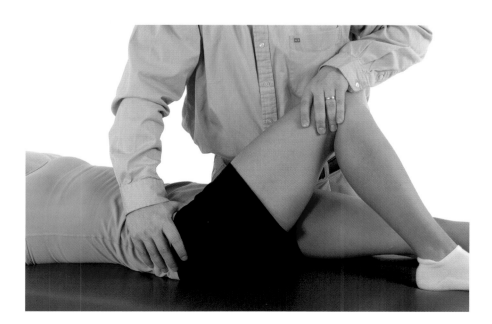

Piriformis

Technique 2

Technique described for the right piriformis muscle.

Patient: Positioned in supine lying with the right hip
flexed to 100° and the right knee flexed to 90°.

Therapist: Standing at the side of the bed.

Action: Stabilize the patient's right innominate with
your left hand and support the distal aspect of their
right tibia and fibula with your right hand and forearm. Adduct and laterally rotate the right hip and
assess the amount of range and the end feel. Both
the stabilizing hand and the hand moving the body
part sense the tension in the muscle and the barrier.
Note the reproduction of any symptoms. Repeat this
test on the contralateral side and compare the two
results.

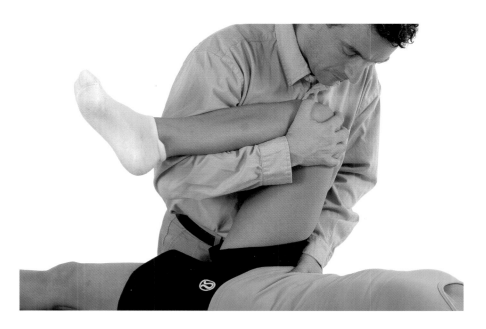

Iliopsoas

Technique described for the right iliopsoas muscle.

Patient: Positioned at the edge of the bed in supine lying with the left hip flexed and the right hip extended over the edge of the bed.

Therapist: Standing at the end of the bed with the patient's left foot supported against the side of the therapist's body.

Action: Stabilize the patient's right anterior superior iliac spine and iliac crest with your right hand. Support the distal aspect of their right femur with your left hand and thigh. Extend, adduct and medially rotate the patient's right hip. Slightly flex the patient's right knee also, to slacken the right sartorius muscle and bias the right iliacus muscle. Monitor the lumbar spine for any changes in the lumbar lordosis. Both the stabilizing hand and the hand moving the body part sense the tension in the muscle and the barrier. Assess the amount of range and the end feel of the right hip and note the reproduction of any symptoms. Repeat this test on the contralateral side and compare the two results.

To assess the psoas, add side flexion of the lumbar spine.

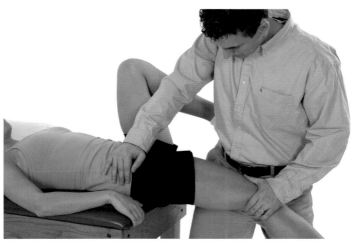

Tensor Fascia Latae

Technique described for the right tensor fascia latae muscle.

Patient: Positioned at the edge of the bed in supine lying with the left hip flexed and the right hip extended over the edge of the bed.

Therapist: Standing at the end of the bed with the patient's left foot supported against the lateral side of the therapist's body.

Action: Stabilize the patient's right anterior superior iliac spine and iliac crest with your right hand. Support the distal aspect of their right femur with your left hand and thigh. To bias the right tensor fascia latae muscle, extend, adduct and laterally rotate the patient's right hip with their knee fully extended.

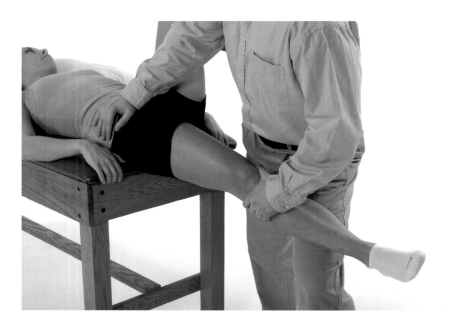

Both the stabilizing hand and the hand moving the body part sense the tension in the muscle and the barrier. Assess the amount of range and the end feel of the right hip and note the reproduction of any symptoms. Repeat this test on the contralateral side and compare the two results.

The action of the tensor fascia latae muscle is similar to that of the gluteus medius (anterior fibers) and the gluteus minimus. To bias the tensor fascia latae muscle and differentiate it, take up the extension component of the combined movements first.

Sartorius

Technique described for the right sartorius muscle.

Patient: Positioned at the edge of the bed in supine lying with the left hip flexed and the right hip extended over the edge of the bed.

Therapist: Standing at the end of the bed with the patient's left foot supported against the lateral side of the therapist's body.

Action: Stabilize the patient's right anterior superior iliac spine and iliac crest with your right hand. Support the distal aspect of their right femur with your left hand and thigh. Extend, adduct and medially rotate the right hip. Fully extend the right knee to slacken the right rectus femoris muscle and bias the right sartorius muscle. Both the stabilizing hand and the hand moving the body part sense the tension in the muscle and the barrier. Assess the amount of range and the end feel of the right hip and note the reproduction of any symptoms. Repeat this test on the contralateral side and compare the two results.

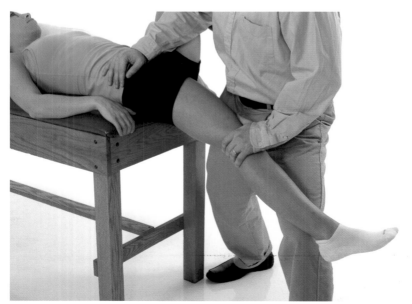

Iliotibial Band

Technique 1 – Modified Ober's Test
Technique described for the right iliotibial band.

Patient: Positioned in left side lying with the left hip flexed and the right knee fully extended.

Therapist: Standing behind the patient with the patient's back against the anterior aspect of the therapist's body.

Action: Stabilize the patient's right iliac crest with your left hand. With your right hand, support the distal aspect of the patient's right femur and right lower leg in a fully extended position. Passively abduct and extend the right hip and then slowly lower it into an adducted position. Both the stabilizing hand and the hand moving the body part sense the tension in the fascia and the barrier. Assess the amount of range and the end feel of the right iliotibial band and note the reproduction of any symptoms. Repeat this test on the contralateral side and compare the two results.

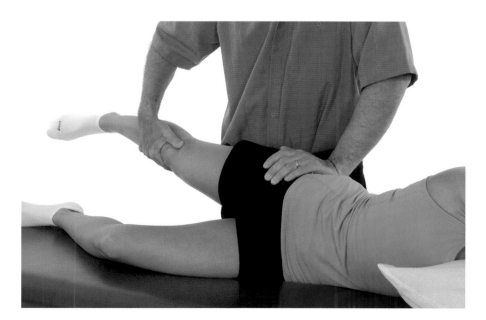

Iliotibial Band

Technique 2 – Modified Ober's Test

Technique described for the right iliotibial band.

Patient: Positioned in left side lying with the left hip flexed and the right knee flexed to 90°.

Therapist: Standing behind the patient with the patient's back against the anterior aspect of the therapist's body.

Action: Stabilize the patient's right iliac crest with your left hand. With your right hand, support the distal aspect of their right femur and right lower leg in a flexed position. Passively abduct and extend the right hip and then slowly lower it into an adducted position. Both the stabilizing hand and the hand moving the body part sense the tension in the fascia and the barrier. Assess the amount of range and the end feel of the right iliotibial band and note the reproduction of any symptoms. Repeat this test on the contralateral side and compare the two results.

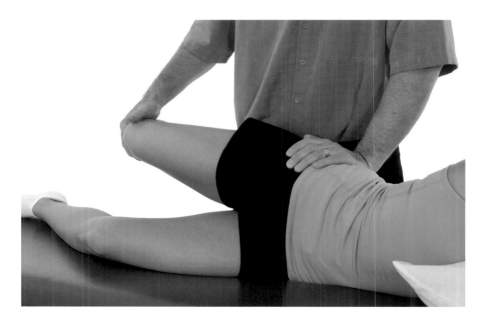

THE KNEE

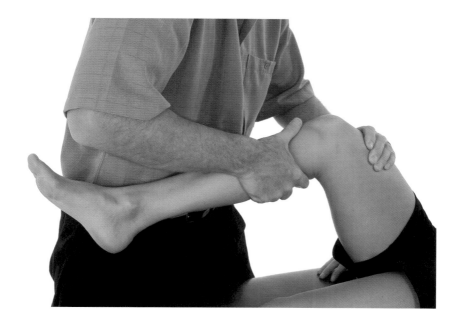

Rectus Femoris

Technique described for the right rectus femoris muscle.

Patient: Positioned at the edge of the bed in supine lying with the left hip flexed and the right hip extended over the edge of the bed.

Therapist: Standing at the end of the bed with the patient's left foot supported against the side of the therapist's body.

Action: Stabilize the patient's right anterior inferior iliac spine and iliac crest with your right hand. Support the distal aspect of their right femur with your left hand. Extend the patient's right hip and flex their right knee to bias the right rectus femoris muscle. Both the stabilizing hand and the hand moving the body part sense the tension in the muscle and the barrier. Assess the amount of range and the end feel of the right knee and note the reproduction of any symptoms. Repeat this test on the contralateral side and compare the two results.

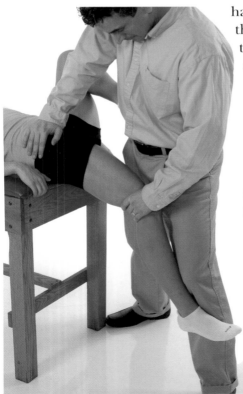

Hamstrings Functional Length Tension Test

Technique 1
Technique described for the right hamstring muscles.

Patient: Positioned in sitting with the lumbar spine positioned in neutral.

Therapist: Standing behind the patient.

Action: Palpate the inferior aspect of the patient's right posterior superior iliac spine with your right thumb and their right sacral base with your left thumb. Instruct the patient to extend their right knee. Note any compensatory movement such as posterior rotation of the pelvis or flexion of the lumbar spine. Assess the amount of range of right knee extension and note any symptom reproduction. Repeat this test on the contralateral side and compare the two results.

Note also the reproduction of any dural symptoms. To differentiate between the neuromeningeal tissue and the muscle, add various sensitizing movements of the spine and lower extremities and note any change in the amount of range, the end feel and the symptoms produced.

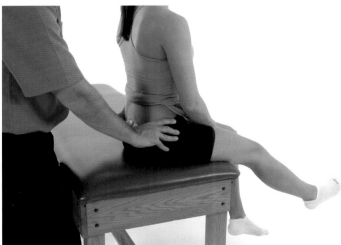

Hamstrings Functional Length Tension Test

Technique 2
Technique described for the right hamstring muscles.

Patient: Positioned in long sitting.

Therapist: Standing at the side of the bed.

Action: Instruct the patient to flex forward at the hip and reach for their toes. Hamstring flexibility is exhausted when you see the lumbar spine flex or the lumbar spine lordosis unwind. Assess the amount of range and note the reproduction of any symptoms.

Note also the reproduction of any dural symptoms. To differentiate between the neuromeningeal tissue and the muscle, add various sensitizing movements of the spine and note any change in the amount of range, the end feel and the symptoms produced.

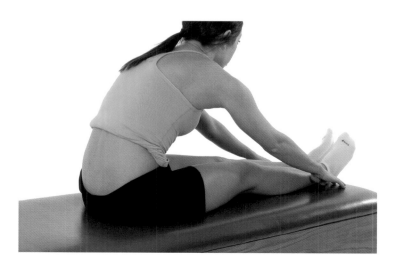

Hamstrings, General

Technique described for the right hamstring muscles.

Patient: Positioned in supine lying.

Therapist: Standing at the side of the bed.

Action: Palpate the patient's right anterior superior iliac spine and iliac crest with your left thumb and index finger. Support the distal aspect of their right tibia and fibula with your right hand. Take the patient's right leg into hip flexion with the knee extended. Hamstring flexibility is exhausted when you feel the right innominate start to rotate posteriorly. Both the stabilizing hand and the hand moving the body part sense the tension in the muscle and the barrier. Assess the amount of range and the end feel of the right leg and note the reproduction of any symptoms. Repeat this test on the contralateral side and compare the two results.

Also note the reproduction of any dural symptoms. To differentiate between the neuromeningeal tissue and the muscle, add various sensitizing movements of the spine and lower extremities and note any change in the amount of range, the end feel and the symptoms produced.

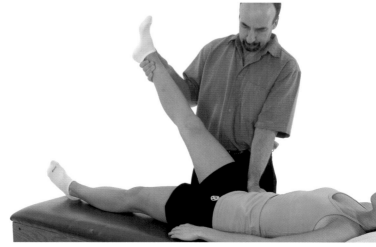

Hamstrings, Medial

Semitendinosus and Semimembranosus
Technique described for the right semitendinosus and right semimembranosus muscles.

Patient: Positioned in supine lying.

Therapist: Standing at the side of the bed.

Action: Palpate the patient's right anterior superior iliac spine and iliac crest with your left thumb and index finger. Support the distal aspect of their right tibia and fibula with your right hand proximal to the right ankle joint. Take the patient's right leg into hip flexion with their knee extended. Add external rotation of the tibia to bias the right semitendinosus and semimembranosus muscles. Flexibility of the semitendinosus and semimembranosus is exhausted when you feel the patient's right innominate start to rotate posteriorly. Both the stabilizing hand and the hand moving the body part sense the tension

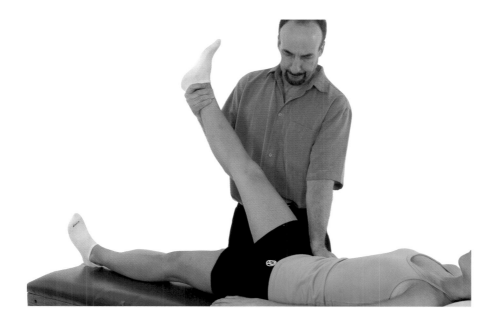

in the muscle and the barrier. Assess the amount of range and the end feel of the right leg and note the reproduction of any symptoms. Repeat this test on the contralateral side and compare the two results.

Also note the reproduction of any dural symptoms. To differentiate between the neuromeningeal tissue and the muscle, add various sensitizing movements of the spine and lower extremities and note any change in the amount of range, the end feel and the symptoms produced.

Hamstrings, Lateral

Biceps Femoris
Technique described for the right biceps femoris muscle.

Patient: Positioned in supine lying.

Therapist: Standing at the side of the bed.

Action: Palpate the patient's right anterior superior iliac spine and iliac crest with your left thumb and index finger. Support the distal aspect of their right tibia and fibula with your right hand proximal to the right ankle joint. Take the patient's right leg into hip flexion with the knee extended. Add internal rotation of the tibia to bias the right biceps femoris muscle. Flexibility of the biceps femoris is exhausted when you feel the patient's right innominate start to rotate posteriorly. Both the stabilizing hand and the hand moving the body part sense the tension in the muscle and the barrier. Assess the amount of range and the end feel of the patient's right leg and

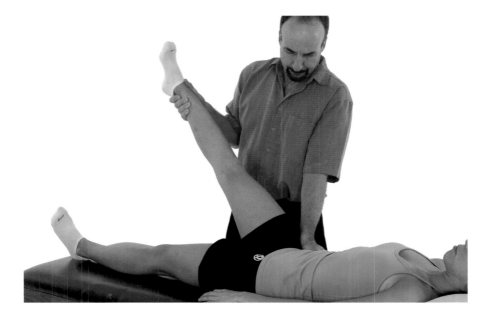

note the reproduction of any symptoms. Repeat this test on the contralateral side and compare the two results.

Also note the reproduction of any dural symptoms. To differentiate between the neuromeningeal tissue and the muscle, add various sensitizing movements of the spine and lower extremities and note any change in the amount of range, the end feel and the symptoms produced.

Gastrocnemius

Technique described for the right gastrocnemius muscle.

Patient: Positioned in supine lying with the right foot extending over the edge of the bed.

Therapist: Standing at the end of the bed.

Action: Support the patient's right knee in full extension with your left hand while supporting the plantar aspect of their right foot with your right hand and forearm. Dorsiflex the patient's right ankle and assess the amount of range and the end feel. Note the reproduction of any symptoms. Repeat this test on the contralateral side and compare the two results.

To bias the medial head of the right gastrocnemius muscle, you can dorsiflex and laterally rotate the ankle and lower leg. To bias the lateral head of the right gastrocnemius, you can dorsiflex and medially rotate the ankle and lower leg. Both the stabilizing hand and the hand moving the body part sense the tension in the muscle and the barrier. Assess the amount of range and the end feel of the right ankle in each of these positions and note the reproduction of any symptoms. Repeat this test on the contralateral side and compare the two results.

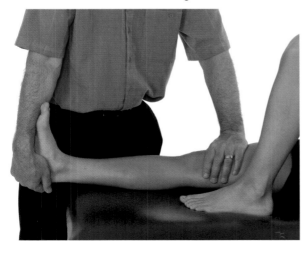

Soleus

Technique 1
Technique described for the right soleus muscle.

Patient: Positioned in supine lying with the right foot extending over the edge of the bed.

Therapist: Standing at the end of the bed.

Action: Support the patient's right knee in flexion with your left hand while supporting the plantar aspect of their right foot with your right hand. Dorsiflex the patient's right ankle and assess the amount of range and the end feel. Note the reproduction of any symptoms. Both the stabilizing hand and the hand moving the body part sense the tension in the muscle and the barrier. Repeat this test on the contralateral side and compare the two results.

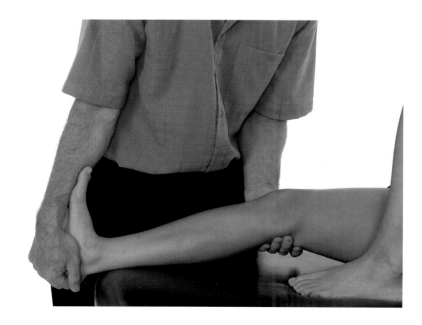

Soleus

Technique 2
Technique described for the right soleus muscle.

Patient: Positioned in sitting with the knees flexed over the edge of the bed.

Therapist: Standing at the end of the bed.

Action: Support the patient's right knee with your left hand while supporting the plantar aspect of their right foot with your right hand and forearm. Dorsiflex the patient's right ankle and assess the amount of range and the end feel. Note the reproduction of any symptoms. Both the stabilizing hand and the hand moving the body part sense the tension in the muscle and the barrier. Repeat this test on the contralateral side and compare the two results.

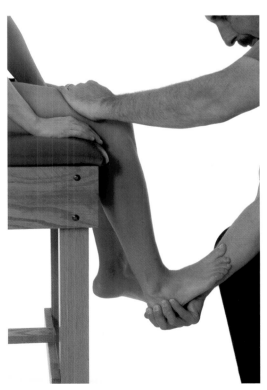

Popliteus

Technique described for the right popliteus muscle.

Patient: Positioned in supine lying.

Therapist: Standing at the side of the bed.

Action: Use your left hand to support the patient's right knee and hip in slight flexion while supporting their right tibia with your right hand and forearm. Externally rotate the patient's right tibia while their right femur is fixed. Both the stabilizing hand and the hand moving the body part sense the tension in the muscle and the barrier. Assess the amount of range and the end feel and note the reproduction of any symptoms. Repeat this test on the contralateral side and compare the two results.

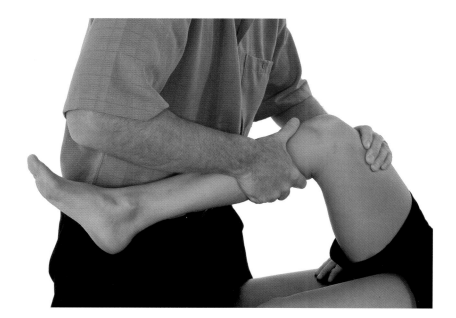

THE FOOT AND ANKLE

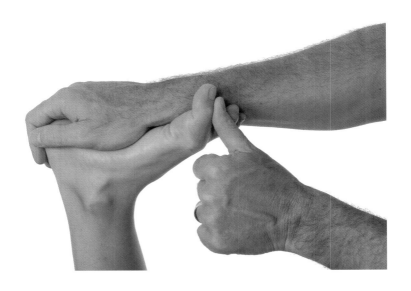

Flexor Hallucis Longus

Technique 1
Technique described for the right flexor hallucis longus muscle.

Patient: Positioned in standing.

Therapist: Kneeling beside the patient's right foot.

Action: Support the anterior aspect of the patient's right ankle with your left hand. With your right hand, extend the patient's right first metatarsophalangeal joint. Both the stabilizing hand and the hand moving the body part sense the tension in the muscle and the barrier. Assess the amount of range and the end feel and note the reproduction of any symptoms. Repeat this test on the contralateral side and compare the two results.

To bias the flexor hallucis longus muscle and differentiate this from tightness in the plantar fascia, you can dorsiflex the patient's ankle by having them bring their knee forward over their foot and then extending the first metatarsophalangeal joint.

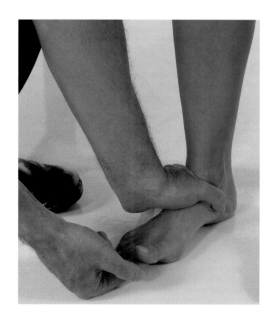

Flexor Hallucis Longus

Technique 2

Technique described for the right flexor hallucis longus muscle.

Patient: Positioned in supine lying with the right foot extending over the edge of the bed.

Therapist: Standing at the end of the bed.

Action: Use your right hand and forearm to support the plantar aspect of the patient's right foot in dorsiflexion while your left hand extends their right first metatarsophalangeal joint. Both the stabilizing hand and the hand moving the body part sense the tension in the muscle and the barrier. Assess the amount of range and the end feel and note the reproduction of any symptoms. Repeat this test on the contralateral side and compare the two results.

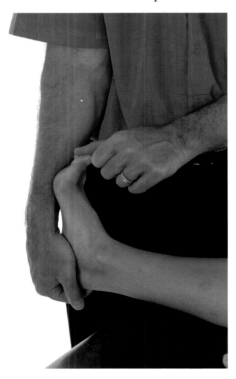

Flexor Hallucis Longus

Technique 3

Technique described for the right flexor hallucis longus muscle.

Patient: Positioned in prone lying with the right knee flexed to 90°.

Therapist: Standing on the right side of the bed.

Action: Use your left hand and forearm to support the plantar aspect of the patient's right foot in dorsiflexion while your right hand extends their right first metatarsophalangeal joint. Both the stabilizing hand and the hand moving the body part sense the tension in the muscle and the barrier. Assess the amount of range and the end feel and note the reproduction of any symptoms. Repeat this test on the contralateral side and compare the two results.

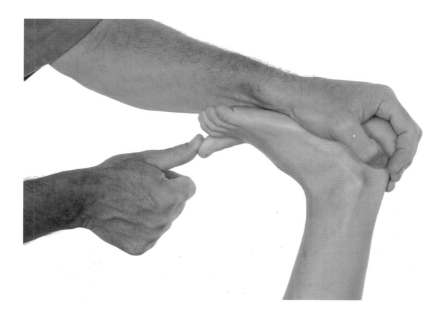

Flexor Hallucis Brevis

Technique 1
Technique described for the right flexor hallucis brevis muscle.

Patient: Positioned in supine lying with the right foot extending over the edge of the bed.

Therapist: Standing at the end of the bed.

Action: Use your left hand to support the dorsal aspect of the patient's right foot in plantarflexion while your right hand extends their right first metatarsophalangeal joint. Both the stabilizing hand and the hand moving the body part sense the tension in the muscle and the barrier. Assess the amount of range and the end feel and note the reproduction of any symptoms. Repeat this test on the contralateral side and compare the two results.

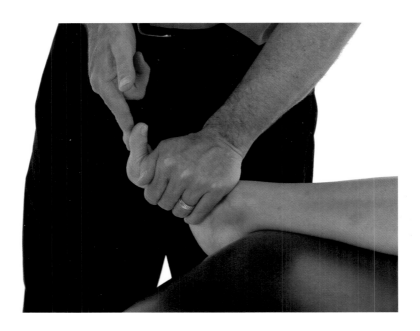

Flexor Hallucis Brevis

Technique 2
Technique described for the right flexor hallucis brevis muscle.

Patient: Positioned in prone lying with the right knee flexed to 90°.

Therapist: Standing at the end of the bed.

Action: Use your left hand to support the dorsal aspect of the patient's right foot in plantarflexion while your right hand extends their right first metatarso-phalangeal joint. Both the stabilizing hand and the hand moving the body part sense the tension in the muscle and the barrier. Assess the amount of range and the end feel and note the reproduction of any symptoms. Repeat this test on the contralateral side and compare the two results.

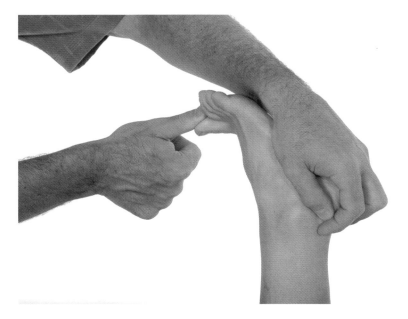

Flexor Digitorum Longus

Technique 1
Technique described for the right flexor digitorum longus muscle.

Patient: Positioned in standing.

Therapist: Kneeling beside the patient's right foot.

Action: Use your left hand to support the anterior aspect of the patient's right ankle while your right fingers extend their right second through fifth metatarsophalangeal joints. Both the stabilizing hand and the hand moving the body part sense the tension in the muscle and the barrier. Assess the amount of range and the end feel and note the reproduction of any symptoms. Repeat this test on the contralateral side and compare the two results.

To bias the flexor digitorum longus muscle and differentiate this from tightness in the plantar fascia, you can dorsiflex the patient's ankle by having them bring their knee forward over their foot and then extending the first metatarsophalangeal joint.

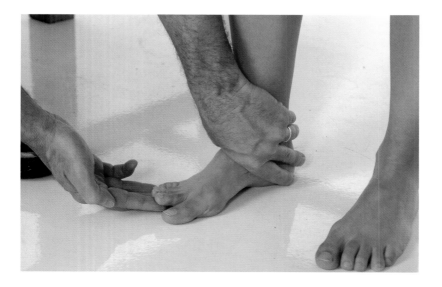

Flexor Digitorum Longus

Technique 2

Technique described for the right flexor digitorum longus muscle.

Patient: Positioned in supine lying with the right foot extending over the edge of the bed.

Therapist: Standing at the end of the bed.

Action: Use your right hand and forearm to support the plantar aspect of the patient's right foot in dorsiflexion while your left thumb extends their right second through fifth metatarsophalangeal joints. Both the stabilizing hand and the hand moving the body part sense the tension in the muscle and the barrier. Assess the amount of range and the end feel and note the reproduction of any symptoms. Repeat this test on the contralateral side and compare the two results.

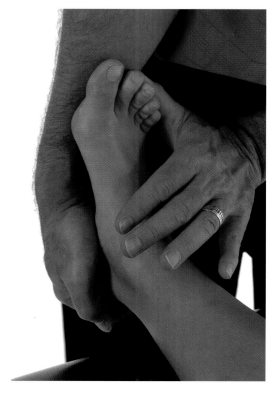

Flexor Digitorum Longus

Technique 3
Technique described for the right flexor digitorum longus muscle.

Patient: Positioned in prone lying with the right knee flexed to 90°.

Therapist: Standing at the end of the bed.

Action: Use your left hand and forearm to support the plantar aspect of the patient's right foot in dorsiflexion while your right fingers extend their right second through fifth metatarsophalangeal joints. Both the stabilizing hand and the hand moving the body part sense the tension in the muscle and the barrier. Assess the amount of range and the end feel and note the reproduction of any symptoms. Repeat this test on the contralateral side and compare the two results.

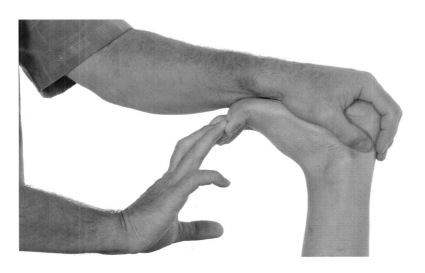

Flexor Digitorum Brevis

Technique 1

Technique described for the right flexor digitorum brevis muscle.

Patient: Positioned in supine lying with the right foot extending over the edge of the bed.

Therapist: Standing at the end of the bed.

Action: Use your left hand to support the dorsal aspect of the patient's right foot in plantarflexion while your right fingers extend their right second through fifth metatarsophalangeal joints. Both the stabilizing hand and the hand moving the body part sense the tension in the muscle and the barrier. Assess the amount of range and the end feel and note the reproduction of any symptoms. Repeat this test on the contralateral side and compare the two results.

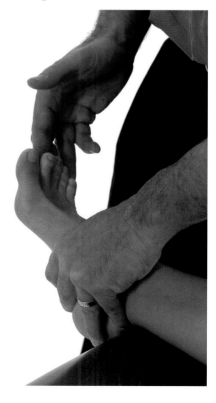

Flexor Digitorum Brevis

Technique 2

Technique described for the right flexor digitorum brevis muscle.

Patient: Positioned in prone lying with the right knee flexed to 90°.

Therapist: Standing at the end of the bed.

Action: Use your left hand to support the dorsal aspect of the patient's right foot in plantarflexion while your right fingers extend their right second through fifth metatarsophalangeal joints. Both the stabilizing hand and the hand moving the body part sense the tension in the muscle and the barrier. Assess the amount of range and the end feel and note the reproduction of any symptoms. Repeat this test on the contralateral side and compare the two results.

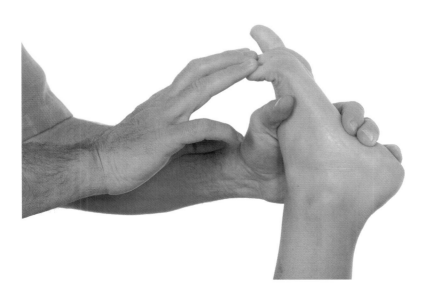

Extensor Hallucis Longus

Technique 1

Technique described for the right extensor hallucis longus muscle.

Patient: Positioned in supine lying with the right foot extending over the edge of the bed.

Therapist: Standing at the end of the bed.

Action: Use your left hand to support the dorsal aspect of the patient's right foot in plantarflexion while your thumb and index finger extend their right first metatarsophalangeal joint. Both the stabilizing hand and the hand moving the body part sense the tension in the muscle and the barrier. Assess the amount of range and the end feel and note the reproduction of any symptoms. Repeat this test on the contralateral side and compare the two results.

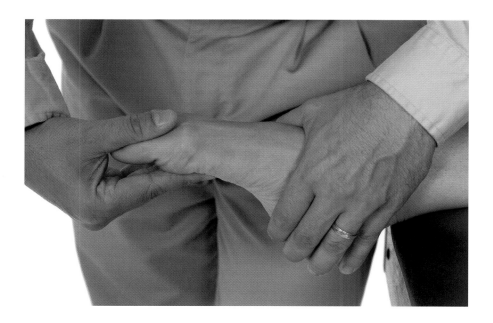

Extensor Hallucis Longus

Technique 2

Technique described for the right extensor hallucis
longus muscle.

Patient: Positioned in prone lying with the right knee
flexed to 90°.

Therapist: Standing at the end of the bed.

Action: Use your left hand to support the dorsal aspect
of the patient's right foot in plantarflexion while
your right thumb flexes their right first metatarsophalangeal joint. Both the stabilizing hand and the
hand moving the body part sense the tension in the
muscle and the barrier. Assess the amount of range
and the end feel and note the reproduction of any
symptoms. Repeat this test on the contralateral side
and compare the two results.

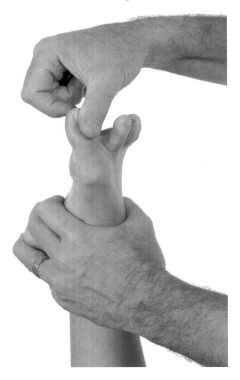

Extensor Hallucis Brevis

Technique 1

Technique described for the right extensor hallucis brevis muscle.

Patient: Positioned in supine lying with the right foot extending over the edge of the bed.

Therapist: Standing at the end of the bed.

Action: Use your right hand and forearm to support the plantar aspect of the patient's right foot in dorsiflexion while your left index finger flexes their right first metatarsophalangeal joint. Both the stabilizing hand and the hand moving the body part sense the tension in the muscle and the barrier. Assess the amount of range and the end feel and note the reproduction of any symptoms. Repeat this test on the contralateral side and compare the two results.

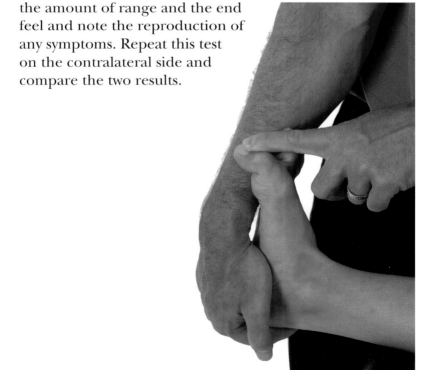

Extensor Hallucis Brevis

Technique 2

Technique described for the right extensor hallucis
brevis muscle.

Patient: Positioned in prone lying with the right knee
flexed to 90°.

Therapist: Standing at the end of the bed.

Action: Use your right hand and forearm to support
the plantar aspect of the patient's right foot in dorsiflexion while your left thumb flexes their right first
metatarsophalangeal joint. Both the stabilizing hand
and the hand moving the body part sense the tension
in the muscle and the barrier. Assess the amount of
range and the end feel and note the reproduction of
any symptoms. Repeat this test on the contralateral
side and compare the two results.

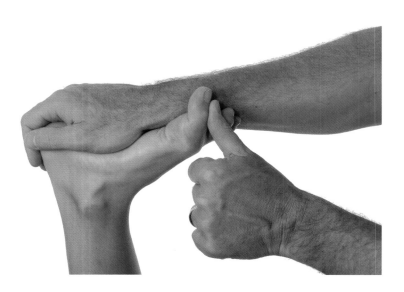

Extensor Digitorum Longus

Technique 1

Technique described for the right extensor digitorum longus muscle.

Patient: Positioned in supine lying with the right foot extending over the edge of the bed.

Therapist: Standing at the end of the bed.

Action: Use your left hand to support the dorsal aspect of the patient's right foot in plantarflexion while your right thumb flexes their right second through fifth metatarsophalangeal joints. Both the stabilizing hand and the hand moving the body part sense the tension in the muscle and the barrier. Assess the amount of range and the end feel and note the reproduction of any symptoms. Repeat this test on the con-tralateral side and compare the two results.

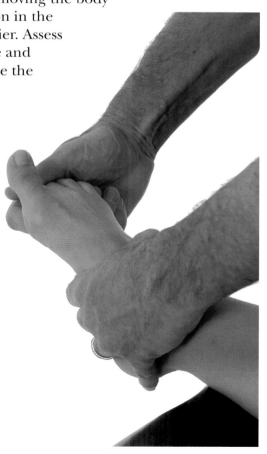

Extensor Digitorum Longus

Technique 2
Technique described for the right extensor digitorum longus muscle.

Patient: Positioned in prone lying with the right knee flexed to 90°.

Therapist: Standing at the end of the bed.

Action: Use your left hand to support the dorsal aspect of the patient's right foot in plantarflexion while your right fingers flex their right second through fifth metatarsophalangeal joints. Both the stabilizing hand and the hand moving the body part sense the tension in the muscle and the barrier. Assess the amount of range and the end feel and note the reproduction of any symptoms. Repeat this test on the contralateral side and compare the two results.

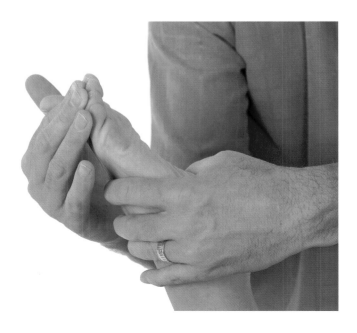

Extensor Digitorum Brevis

Technique 1

Technique described for the right extensor digitorum
brevis muscle.

Patient: Positioned in supine lying with the right foot
 extending over the edge of the bed.

Therapist: Standing at the end of the bed.

Action: Use your right hand and forearm to support
 the plantar aspect of the patient's right foot in
 dorsiflexion while your left thumb flexes their right
 second through fifth metatarsophalangeal joints.
 Both the stabilizing hand and the hand moving the
 body part sense the tension in the muscle and the
 barrier. Assess the amount of range and the end feel
 and note the reproduction of any symptoms. Repeat
 this test on the
 contralateral side
 and compare the
 two results.

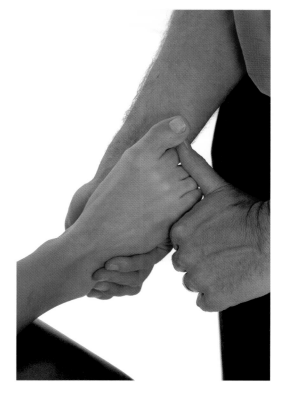

Extensor Digitorum Brevis

Technique 2
Technique described for the right extensor digitorum
brevis muscle.

Patient: Positioned in prone lying with the right knee
flexed to 90°.

Therapist: Standing at the end of the bed.

Action: Use your left hand and forearm to support the
plantar aspect of the patient's right foot in dorsiflexion while your right fingers flex their right second
through fifth metatarsophalangeal joints. Both the
stabilizing hand and the hand moving the body part
sense the tension in the muscle and the barrier.
Assess the amount of range and the end feel and note
the reproduction of any symptoms. Repeat this test
on the contralateral side and compare the two results.

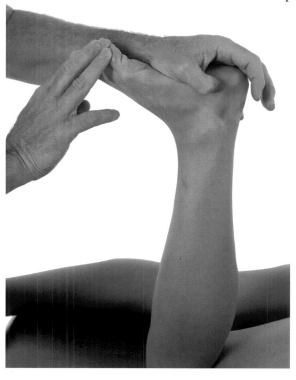

Tibialis Posterior

Technique 1
Technique described for the right tibialis posterior muscle.

Patient: Positioned in supine lying with the right foot extending over the edge of the bed.

Therapist: Standing at the end of the bed.

Action: Use your left hand to stabilize the anterior aspect of the patient's distal right lower leg. Your right hand and forearm support the plantar aspect of the patient's right hindfoot and midfoot in dorsiflexion and everts the patient's right midfoot. Both the stabilizing hand and the hand moving the body part sense the tension in the muscle and the barrier. Assess the amount of range and the end feel and note the reproduction of any symptoms. Repeat this test on the contralateral side and compare the two results.

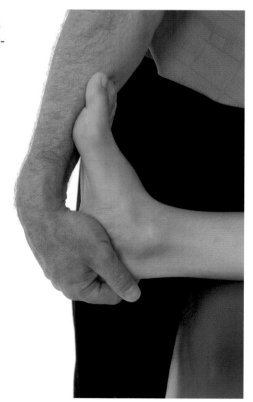

Tibialis Posterior

Technique 2
Technique described for the right tibialis posterior muscle.

Patient: Positioned in prone lying with the right knee flexed to 90°.

Therapist: Standing on the right side of the bed.

Action: Use your right hand to support the distal aspect of the patient's right lower leg. Your left hand holds the hindfoot and midfoot in dorsiflexion and everts the patient's right midfoot. Both the stabilizing hand and the hand moving the body part sense the tension in the muscle and the barrier. Assess the amount of range and the end feel and note the reproduction of any symptoms. Repeat this test on the contralateral side and compare the two results.

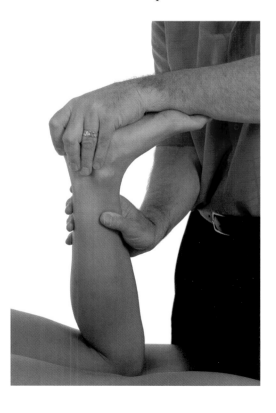

Tibialis Anterior

Technique 1

Technique described for the right tibialis anterior muscle.

Patient: Positioned in supine lying with the right foot extending over the edge of the bed.

Therapist: Standing at the end of the bed.

Action: Use your left hand to support the proximal aspect of the patient's right lower leg. Your right hand supports the dorsal aspect of the patient's right hindfoot and midfoot in plantarflexion and everts the right midfoot. Both the stabilizing hand and the hand moving the body part sense the tension in the muscle and the barrier. Assess the amount of range and the end feel and note the reproduction of any symptoms. Repeat this test on the contralateral side and compare the two results.

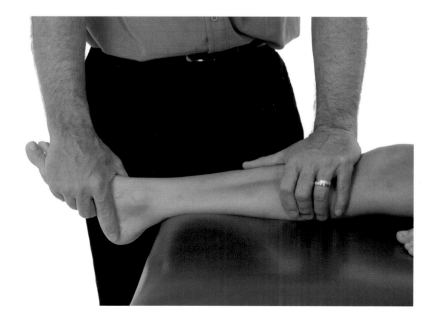

Tibialis Anterior

Technique 2
Technique described for the right tibialis anterior muscle.

Patient: Positioned in prone lying with the right knee
   flexed to 90°.

Therapist: Standing on the right side of the bed.

Action: Use your right hand and forearm to support the
   proximal aspect of the patient's right lower leg. Your
   left hand holds the right hindfoot and midfoot in plantarflexion and everts the patient's right midfoot. Both
   the stabilizing hand and the hand moving the body
   part sense the tension in the muscle and the barrier.
   Assess the amount of range and the end feel and note
   the reproduction of any symptoms. Repeat this test on
   the contralateral side and compare the two results.

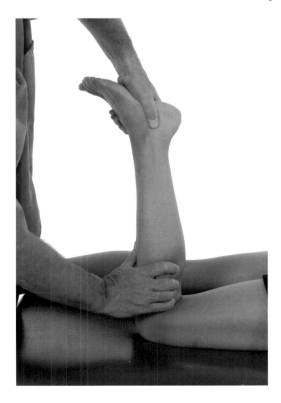

Peroneus Longus and Peroneus Brevis

Technique 1

Technique described for the right peroneus longus and peroneus brevis muscles.

Patient: Positioned in supine lying with the right foot extending over the edge of the bed.

Therapist: Standing at the end of the bed.

Action: Use your left hand to support the plantar aspect of the patient's right hindfoot in dorsiflexion. Your right hand holds the patient's right midfoot and forefoot in plantarflexion and inversion. Both the stabilizing hand and the hand moving the body part sense the tension in the muscle and the barrier. Assess the amount of range and the end feel and note the reproduction of any symptoms. Repeat this test on the contralateral side and compare the two results.

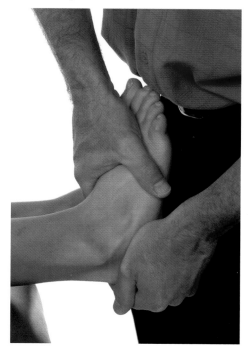

Peroneus Longus and Peroneus Brevis

Technique 2
Technique described for the right peroneus longus and peroneus brevis muscles.

Patient: Positioned in prone lying with the right knee flexed to 90°.

Therapist: Standing on the right side of the bed.

Action: Use your left hand to hold the patient's right hindfoot in dorsiflexion while your right hand holds their midfoot and forefoot in plantarflexion and inversion. Both the stabilizing hand and the hand moving the body part sense the tension in the muscle and the barrier. Assess the amount of range and the end feel and note the reproduction of any symptoms. Repeat this test on the contralateral side and compare the two results.

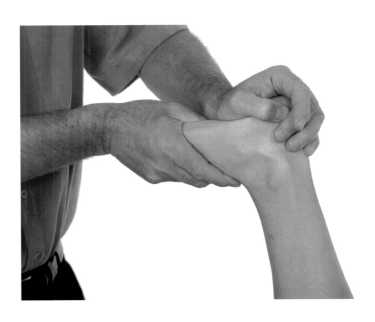

Peroneus Tertius

Technique 1

Technique described for the right peroneus tertius muscle.

Patient: Positioned in supine lying with the right foot extending over the edge of the bed.

Therapist: Standing at the end of the bed.

Action: Use your right hand to support the distal aspect of the patient's right tibia and fibula. Your left hand holds the patient's right hindfoot and midfoot in plantarflexion and then takes the midfoot into inversion. Both the stabilizing hand and the hand moving the body part sense the tension in the muscle and the barrier. Assess the amount of range and the end feel and note the reproduction of any symptoms. Repeat this test on the contralateral side and compare the two results.

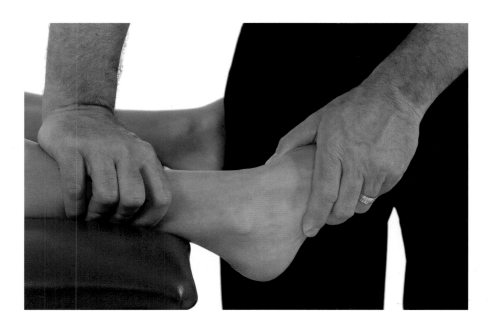

Peroneus Tertius

Technique 2

Technique described for the right peroneus tertius muscle.

Patient: Positioned in prone lying with the right knee flexed to 90°.

Therapist: Standing on the right side of the bed.

Action: Your left hand supports the distal aspect of the patient's right tibia and fibula. Your right hand holds the patient's right hindfoot and midfoot in plantar-flexion and then takes the midfoot into inversion. Both the stabilizing hand and the hand moving the body part sense the tension in the muscle and the barrier. Assess the amount of range and the end feel and note the reproduction of any symptoms. Repeat this test on the contralateral side and compare the two results.

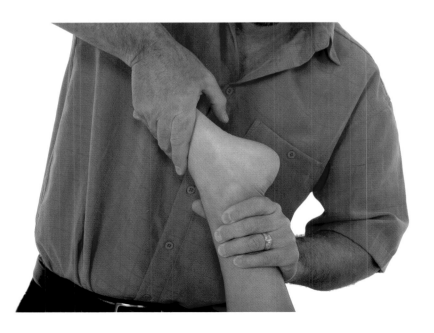

References

Butler, D. 1991. *Mobilization of the Nervous System.* New York: Churchill Livingstone.

Butler, D. 2000. *The Sensitive Nervous System.* Adelaide, Australia: Noigroup Publications.

Evjenth, O. 1993. *Muscle Stretching in Manual Therapy: A Clinical Manual – The Extremities,* Vol. 1. Alfta, Sweden: Alfta Rehab.

Evjenth, O., and J. Hamberg. 1993. *Muscle Stretching in Manual Therapy: A Clinical Manual – The Extremities.* Alfta, Sweden: Alfta Rehab.

Magee, D. 2014. *Orthopedic Physical Assessment.* 6th ed. New York: Elsevier Saunders.

Peterson-Kendall, F., E. Kendall-McCreary, P. Geise-Provance, M. McIntyre-Rodgers, and W.A. Romani. 2005. *Muscles: Testing and Function with Posture and Pain.* 5th ed. Baltimore, Md.: Lippincott, Williams and Wilkins.

Sahrmann, S.A. 2002. *Diagnosis and Treatment of Movement Impairment Syndromes.* St. Louis, Mo.: Mosby.

About the Authors

Paolo Sanzo is a physiotherapist at the Victoriaville Physiotherapy Centre in Thunder Bay, Ontario. He is an assistant professor in the School of Kinesiology at Lakehead University and at the Northern Ontario School of Medicine. He is also an instructor and examiner with the Orthopaedic Division of the Canadian Physiotherapy Association.

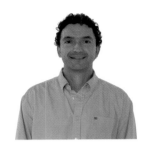

Murray MacHutchon is a physiotherapist at Pembina Physiotherapy and Sports Injury Clinic in Winnipeg, Manitoba. He is also an instructor and examiner with the Orthopaedic Division of the Canadian Physiotherapy Association.

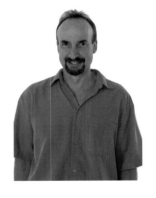

Courses

The authors provide courses in the following areas:
- Length Tension Testing of the Upper and Lower Quadrants
- Muscle Energy
- Release of the Pelvic and Thoracic Outlets
- Understanding Headaches, Facial Pain and the Cranioverte-bral Joint Region
- Assessment and Treatment of Cervicogenic Headaches
- The Cervicothoracic Junction
- The Thoracolumbar Junction
- Sport Taping
- Neuromuscular Facilitative Taping

If you are interested in hosting a course, please do not hesitate to contact us at www.activepotentialrehab.com.